SILVERCORE FITNESS

SENIOR WALL PILATES

How to Age Gracefully, Increase Flexibility, and Maintain Balance Use a Wall to Defy Father Time

This book was professionally typeset on Reedsy.
Find out more at reedsy.com

Contents

1

Introduction

Embracing the Power of Wall Pilates

Welcome to a journey that transcends the boundaries of age and defies the notion that time dictates our vitality. In the following pages, we invite you to explore the transformative world of Wall Pilates – a practice that goes beyond exercise, reaching into the very core of graceful aging and holistic well-being.

Picture this: a room adorned with simplicity, a supportive wall by your side, and the gentle guidance of Pilates principles weaving through your movements. This is not just a workout; it's an embrace of the power that lies within you, waiting to be awakened.

Why Wall Pilates?

In a world filled with fitness trends and fads, Wall Pilates stands out as a timeless companion on your journey to better health. It's not about pushing limits or chasing after unattainable ideals. Instead, it's a celebration of your unique journey, meeting you exactly where you are.

As we embark on this exploration, keep in mind that Wall Pilates isn't reserved for the seasoned fitness enthusiast. It's an open invitation to anyone seeking a path to increased mobility, improved balance, and the joy of pain-free movement – especially our beloved seniors, who deserve every opportunity to savor the richness of life at every stage.

What Awaits You?

This book is more than just words on paper; it's a guide crafted with care to empower you in your Wall Pilates journey. We'll unravel the principles that form the foundation, guide you through the initial steps, and witness together the remarkable stories of individuals whose lives have been touched by the simple yet profound power of Wall Pilates.

2

The Foundation of Wall Pilates

Welcome to the cornerstone of your Wall Pilates journey! In this chapter, we're about to lay the groundwork for a transformative experience that goes beyond exercise – it's about building a foundation for graceful aging, increased mobility, and a life filled with pain-free movement.

The Core Principles of Wall Pilates

Imagine your body as a finely tuned instrument, and the principles of Wall Pilates as the notes that create a harmonious melody. We're talking about core strength that goes beyond the surface, breathing that becomes a rhythm for every movement, and alignment that brings a symphony of balance into your life.

Let's Dive In:

1. The Importance of Core Strength

We often hear about the core, but here, we're going to unravel its profound significance. Your core isn't just about six-pack abs; it's the powerhouse that supports your spine, enhances stability and is the secret ingredient to fluid, controlled movement.

2. Understanding the Breath-work

Ever thought of breathing as a fundamental aspect of fitness? In Wall Pilates, each breath is a cue, guiding your movements and fostering a deep mind-body connection. We'll explore how mindful breathing not only energizes your body but also relaxes your mind, setting the stage for a transformative experience.

3. The Role of Alignment

Imagine your body in perfect alignment – a posture that not only exudes confidence but also minimizes the risk of injury. In this section, we'll delve into the subtle nuances of alignment, understanding how proper positioning can be a game-changer in your journey to pain-free movement.

The Benefits of Wall Pilates

Now that we've laid the groundwork, let's explore the exciting rewards that await you on this Wall Pilates adventure.

Discover:

1. Enhanced Posture and Balance

Picture yourself standing tall, shoulders back, and a newfound sense of poise. Wall Pilates works wonders for your posture, promoting a natural alignment that extends beyond the studio into your daily life. Improved balance becomes not just a goal but a delightful side effect.

2. Increased Flexibility and Strength

Flexibility isn't just for gymnasts; it's a key ingredient for a body that moves with ease. Through carefully curated exercises, Wall Pilates invites flexibility into your life, complemented by newfound strength that empowers you in ways you might not have imagined.

3. Pain Relief and Overall Wellness

Bid farewell to those persistent aches and pains. Wall Pilates isn't just about the workout; it's a holistic approach to well-being. We'll uncover how these gentle movements can alleviate pain, improve circulation, and contribute to your overall physical and mental wellness.

And Now a Tale of Transformation:

Jane's Journey to Pain-Free Movement

Jane, a vibrant senior in her early seventies, had always been active and full of life. However, as the years passed, she began experiencing nagging joint pain, particularly in her knees and lower back. The pain was taking a toll on her active lifestyle and overall well-being.

Determined to regain her pain-free movement, Jane embarked on a journey into the world of Wall Pilates. Her first introduction to Wall Pilates was through a local community center that offered specialized classes for seniors, including those dealing with pain.

Her initial experience was guided by Emily, a Wall Pilates instructor who had a deep understanding of pain management. The class started with gentle warm-up exercises that were specifically designed to alleviate joint discomfort. Jane felt immediate relief as her body began to loosen up.

As Jane moved through the various Wall Pilates exercises with the support of the wall, she was amazed at how the practice targeted the source of her pain.

Emily emphasized proper alignment and posture, which helped relieve the pressure on Jane's joints.

One exercise that significantly impacted Jane's pain was a modified version of the classic Pilates hundred exercise. Using the wall for support, she could engage her core and strengthen her abdominal muscles without straining her lower back. The relief was palpable.

Over time, Jane's commitment to her Wall Pilates practice paid off. She began to experience a gradual reduction in pain, and her flexibility improved. As she continued to strengthen her core and improve her posture, the chronic discomfort that had once plagued her started to subside.

Jane shared her transformation, saying, "Wall Pilates has been a game-changer for me. It's not just about relieving pain; it's about reclaiming my active lifestyle. I can now enjoy my daily walks, gardening, and playing with my grandkids without the constant discomfort."

Jane's story underscores the power of Wall Pilates in pain management for seniors. It highlights the tailored approach to pain relief that Wall Pilates offers and how it can significantly improve the quality of life for those like Jane. Her experience serves as a testament to the effectiveness of Wall Pilates in providing a path to pain-free movement and enhanced overall well-being.

So, whether you're a curious beginner or someone seeking a fresh approach to wellness, fasten your seat belt as we dive into the heart of Wall Pilates. Let's embrace the power it holds – a power that allows us to age with grace, move with ease, and revel in the timeless dance of mind and body.

Welcome to a world where the wall is not just a support; it's a companion in your journey towards embracing the ageless you.

3

Preparing for Your Wall Pilates Journey

Welcome to the prelude of your Wall Pilates adventure! In this chapter, we're not just preparing your body; we're setting the stage for a journey that will empower you to discover newfound strength, resilience, and a profound connection between your mind and body. So, grab your enthusiasm, and let's dive into the essential preparations for your Wall Pilates journey.

Evaluating Your Mobility and Balance

Before we embark on this exciting journey, let's take a moment to understand where you are on the mobility and balance spectrum. It's not about comparison; it's about creating a road map tailored to your unique needs.

Guiding Steps:

1. Self-Assessment Tools

We'll introduce simple self-assessment tools to gauge your current mobility and balance. No need for complicated gadgets — just a willingness to explore your body's capabilities.

2. Setting Realistic Goals

Together, we'll establish realistic goals based on your self-assessment. Whether it's improving flexibility, enhancing balance, or reducing discomfort, your goals will shape your Wall Pilates journey.

3. The Importance of Patience

Patience is your steadfast companion in this preparation phase. Understand that progress takes time, and each step forward is a victory worth celebrating.

Mental Preparation and Mindset

Now, let's shift our focus to the mental aspect of your Wall Pilates journey. Your mindset is a powerful tool, and cultivating the right one will propel you toward success.

Nurturing Your Mindset:

1. The Power of Positivity

We'll explore the impact of a positive mindset on your journey. Positivity isn't just about smiling; it's about approaching challenges with optimism and resilience.

2. Visualizing Your Success

Visualization is a potent technique. Together, we'll envision your success in Wall Pilates, creating a mental image of the vibrant, mobile, and balanced version of yourself.

3. Staying Motivated

Motivation is the heartbeat of any journey. Discover techniques to keep that motivation alive, even on days when the wall seems a bit higher.

A Senior's Initial Doubts and Later Success:

Anna, a senior in her late sixties, had always been mindful of her health. She had tried various exercise programs throughout her life but had never considered Pilates, let alone Wall Pilates. Her initial doubts were rooted in the fear of the unknown. She had heard about Wall Pilates from a friend who had experienced remarkable improvements in flexibility and strength, but Anna remained skeptical.

What worried Anna the most were the preconceived notions she had about Pilates – that it was for the young and fit, and it involved challenging and potentially painful exercises. The idea of hanging upside down from a wall was far from appealing. However, her friend's enthusiasm and visible results were hard to ignore.

Anna's journey into Wall Pilates began with trepidation. She was reassured by her friend that Wall Pilates was gentle and accessible for seniors, which eventually convinced her to give it a try.

She attended her first Wall Pilates class with a mix of curiosity and skepticism. The instructor, Michael, recognized the apprehension in the faces of many newcomers, including Anna. He began the class by addressing the common doubts and questions, making everyone feel at ease.

The initial exercises were designed to be comfortable and gentle. Anna realized that Wall Pilates wasn't about hanging upside down but about using the wall as a supportive tool for a wide range of exercises. As she followed Michael's guidance, she felt the wall providing stability and balance, something she had not expected.

The breathing techniques and mindfulness introduced during the class were transformative for Anna. She began to understand that Wall Pilates wasn't just about physical fitness but also mental well-being. It allowed her to be present in the moment and find a sense of calm.

As the class progressed, Anna's initial doubts began to wane. She found the exercises challenging but not overwhelming. By the end of the class, she felt a sense of accomplishment, and her skepticism had turned into curiosity and enthusiasm.

Anna's Wall Pilates journey continued, and she soon experienced noticeable improvements in her flexibility, posture, and core strength. Her initial doubts had given way to confidence and a newfound appreciation for this gentle yet effective practice.

Anna shares her transformation, saying, "I was once a skeptic, but Wall Pilates has opened a door to a healthier and more balanced life. It's a reminder that it's never too late to try something new and experience personal growth."

Anna's story exemplifies the common doubts and misconceptions many seniors may have about Wall Pilates. It highlights how a supportive instructor and the gentle nature of Wall Pilates can dispel these doubts and lead to surprising success and personal growth. Her narrative serves as a reassuring example of how seniors can overcome initial skepticism and find joy in exploring a new form of fitness.

As you prepare for your Wall Pilates journey, remember that every small effort counts. This chapter lays the groundwork for a holistic approach that encompasses not only the physical but also the mental aspects of your well-being. So, are you ready to set the stage for your Wall Pilates adventure? Let's dive in and lay the foundation for a journey that's uniquely yours.

4

Getting Started with Wall Pilates

Hey Pilates beginner! It's time to take the plunge and dive into the invigorating world of Wall Pilates. In this chapter, we're not just dipping our toes; we're cannon-balling into a pool of rejuvenation, mobility, and delightful movement. So, roll out your exercise mat, find a cozy spot near the wall, and let's kick off your Wall Pilates journey!

Choosing the Right Wall Pilates Space

Before we get into the nitty-gritty of exercises, let's talk about setting the stage. Your environment plays a crucial role in creating a Pilates haven.

Crafting Your Space:

1. Creating a Safe and Comfortable Environment

Your space should be your sanctuary. We'll explore how to ensure a safe and comfortable atmosphere, free from distractions and hazards.

2. Equipment and Props

You don't need a Pilates studio at home. Discover the minimal equipment and props that can elevate your experience – the wall being your primary companion.

3. The Role of a Supportive Wall

Spoiler alert – the wall isn't just a backdrop; it's your ally. Learn how the wall becomes the cornerstone of your practice, offering support and stability.

Your First Wall Pilates Session

Now, let's roll up our sleeves and get moving! Your first session is like the opening scene of a captivating movie – full of anticipation and excitement.

Initiating Your Pilates Adventure:

1. Warm-up and Breathing Exercises

Every good Pilates session begins with a warm-up that not only primes your muscles but also introduces you to the breath work. We'll explore the art of gentle warm-ups and rhythmic breathing to kick-start your journey.

2. Essential Beginner Poses and Stretches

Get ready for a repertoire of beginner-friendly poses and stretches. From toe-tapping exercises to gentle twists, these movements lay the foundation for the intricate dance of Wall Pilates.

3. Overcoming Initial Discomfort

Here's a secret – discomfort is a sign of growth. We'll discuss common challenges newcomers face and how to overcome them, ensuring your initiation into Wall Pilates is smooth sailing.

John's First Experience with Wall Pilates:

John, a 68-year-old retiree, had always been curious about alternative forms of exercise, but he had never ventured far from traditional gym workouts. However, when he began experiencing joint pain and stiffness, he knew he needed a change in his fitness routine. That's when a friend recommended Wall Pilates.

His first experience with Wall Pilates was marked by curiosity and a hint of skepticism. He walked into the well-lit Pilates studio and was greeted by the calming presence of the instructor, Sarah. She had an aura of confidence that immediately put him at ease.

The studio was furnished with the necessary equipment, including yoga mats, resistance bands, and, of course, a wall. John had seen some basic Wall Pilates exercises online, but he wasn't quite sure what to expect.

The class started with a gentle warm-up. Sarah guided the participants through a series of controlled breathing exercises and basic stretches. John noticed that the breathing techniques played a significant role in keeping the class centered and focused.

Then came the Wall Pilates poses. John used the wall for support as he carefully followed the instructor's guidance. The wall, he found, was a reassuring presence, allowing him to maintain balance and alignment during the exercises.

One of the poses involved a gentle stretch that targeted the muscles along his spine. John could feel the tension in his back slowly dissipating. As he moved through the poses, he was pleasantly surprised by the level of challenge and the focus on core strength.

However, it was the final relaxation and mindfulness segment of the class that truly struck a chord with John. Sarah asked the class to lie on their mats, close their eyes, and breathe deeply. She encouraged them to let go of their worries and be present in the moment. John had never experienced this level of mental relaxation in a fitness class.

As the class concluded, John felt a sense of calm, improved flexibility, and an unusual lightness in his body. He was intrigued and excited to explore Wall Pilates further.

John reflects on his first experience, saying, "I entered that studio with a bit of doubt, but I walked out feeling rejuvenated. Wall Pilates offered me something different, not just physically, but mentally as well. It was a unique and holistic approach to fitness that I had been missing all these years."

John's initial encounter with Wall Pilates reflects the curiosity and apprehension that many newcomers feel. It emphasizes the calming and holistic aspects of the practice that go beyond physical exercise. His story serves as an example of how Wall Pilates can surprise and inspire individuals, introducing them to a new dimension of well-being and fitness.

As you prepare for your inaugural Wall Pilates session, remember that every movement is a step toward increased mobility and a healthier, happier you. So, are you ready to embrace the wall as your Pilates partner? Let's embark on this exciting journey, one pose at a time!

5

Building a Strong Foundation

Hello again, Pilates Explorer! Now that you've dipped your toes into the refreshing waters of Wall Pilates, it's time to build a foundation that will withstand the test of time. In this chapter, we're laying the bricks for a resilient, powerhouse core and exploring the secrets to a posture that radiates confidence. So, grab your Pilates mat, find your wall, and let's fortify that foundation!

Understanding the Core: It's More Than Just Abs

In the world of Pilates, the term "core" isn't just a fitness buzzword – it's the epicenter of your strength and stability.

Embarking on Core Exploration:

1. Deep Dive into Core Muscles

Get ready for a journey beneath the surface as we explore the intricate web of muscles that make up your core. Spoiler alert: it's more than just the six-pack!

2. The Role of Core in Stability

Imagine your core as the anchor holding a ship steady in a storm. We'll delve into how a strong core enhances stability, not just during Pilates but in your daily activities.

3. **Building Core Strength Gradually**:

Rome wasn't built in a day, and neither is a robust core. Discover gentle exercises designed to progressively build strength, ensuring a solid foundation for your Pilates practice.

Breathing Life into Your Movements

Remember, Pilates is not just a physical endeavor; it's a dance between breath and movement.

Unlocking the Power of Breath:

1. Connecting Breath with Movement

We'll revisit the rhythmic dance of breath and movement, understanding how synchronized breathing enhances the effectiveness of your Pilates poses.

2. Creating Mind-Body Harmony

Breath isn't just oxygen; it's a conduit for mindfulness. Learn how conscious breathing fosters a deep connection between your mind and body, transforming your Pilates practice into a meditative journey.

3. Applying Breath to Specific Exercises:

Breath isn't a one-size-fits-all concept. We'll tailor breathing techniques to specific exercises, amplifying their impact on your core strength and overall well-being.

Perfecting Posture: The Elixir of Confidence

Picture this: a posture that exudes confidence and grace. Now, let's make that image a reality.

Crafting an Upright Stance:

1. Understanding the Elements of Good Posture

What does good posture entail? We'll dissect the elements of a proper stance, from head to toe, and explore why it matters beyond aesthetics.

2. Incorporating Wall Support

The wall isn't just a bystander; it's your silent partner in achieving optimal posture. Discover how the wall becomes your guide, providing support for a spine that stands tall and proud.

3. Posture Exercises for Daily Life

Pilates isn't confined to the mat. We'll explore exercises that seamlessly integrate into your daily routine, ensuring your newfound posture isn't left behind when you step off the mat.

Case Study: Journey to Improved Posture

Maria, a vibrant senior in her late sixties, had always been a go-getter. She had a career that kept her on her feet and was an avid traveler, exploring different corners of the world. However, as the years went by, Maria noticed a significant change – her posture was deteriorating.

Years of hunching over her desk and the wear and tear from her adventures were taking their toll. Maria's once-upright posture was now slightly slouched, causing discomfort and affecting her overall self-confidence.

She decided to act and seek a solution that would help her regain the posture she once had. That's when she discovered Wall Pilates.

Maria's first Wall Pilates class was a revelation. She realized how her poor posture had been contributing to her discomfort and pain. The instructor explained the significance of a strong core, proper alignment, and the role of the wall in helping seniors like Maria regain their posture.

As she started her Wall Pilates journey, the changes were gradual but noticeable. The wall provided the necessary support and helped her maintain proper alignment during exercises. Maria was determined to regain her upright posture, so she practiced regularly, integrating Wall Pilates into her daily routine.

After several months of consistent practice, Maria experienced a significant transformation. Her posture improved, and she felt taller and more confident. The chronic discomfort she used to feel in her neck and back had diminished. Her friends and family noticed the change too, often commenting on how youthful and energetic she looked.

Maria shares her experience, saying, "Wall Pilates has been a game-changer for me. It's not just about looking better; it's about feeling better. I have my confidence back, and I can continue to explore the world with a strong, upright posture."

Maria's story serves as a testament to the effectiveness of Wall Pilates in improving posture and enhancing one's self-esteem. It demonstrates that, with dedication and the right techniques, even long-standing issues like poor posture can be addressed and improved in a safe and sustainable manner.

Maria's experience with Wall Pilates and her remarkable improvement in posture aligns with several studies that have explored the positive impact of Pilates on posture and alignment in seniors. One such study, conducted by Kloubec, JA (2011, Muscles Ligaments Tendons J. Apr-Jun; 1(2): 61–66.) found the exercises are designed to increase muscle strength and endurance, as well as flexibility and to improve posture and balance. Maria's journey reflects the real-world application of the principles discussed in this study.

As you dive into Chapter 4, remember that building a strong foundation isn't just about muscles and bones; it's about creating a resilient base for a life filled with mobility and confidence. So, are you ready to fortify your Pilates fortress? Let's lay those foundation stones for a powerhouse core and a posture that radiates strength!

6

Enhancing Balance and Coordination

Well done, Pilates adventurer! We've built a solid foundation; now, let's set sail into the seas of balance and coordination. In this chapter, we'll dance on the tightrope of equilibrium, exploring how Wall Pilates becomes not just a workout but a graceful performance of stability and coordination. Ready to waltz with your balance and pirouette with coordination? Let's dive in!

The Dance of Balance: Finding Your Center

Imagine standing tall and steady, a tree rooted firmly against the wind. That's the essence of balance in Pilates.

Discovering Your Center:

1. Understanding the Center of Gravity

Ever wonder why a tightrope walker carries a pole? It's all about the center of gravity. We'll explore how finding your center becomes the key to mastering balance in Wall Pilates.

2. Engaging Core for Stability

Your core isn't just for show; it's your anchor. We'll delve into how activating your core muscles enhances stability, laying the groundwork for graceful and controlled movements.

3. Progressive Balance Exercises

From simple weight shifts to more advanced poses, we'll embark on a series of balance exercises designed to challenge and strengthen your stabilizing muscles gradually.

Coordination: The Choreography of Movement

Pilates is not just about isolated poses; it's a symphony of movements that require seamless coordination.

Harmonizing Your Movements:

1. Mind-Body Connection in Action

Coordination isn't just about moving limbs; it's a conversation between your mind and body. We'll explore how cultivating this connection transforms your Pilates practice into a rhythmic dance.

2. Sequential Movements for Fluidity

Like a well-choreographed dance routine, Pilates exercises often involve a sequence of movements. We'll unravel the secrets of performing these sequences with grace and precision.

3. Integrating Wall Support

The wall isn't a mere bystander; it's your dance partner. Discover how the wall provides subtle guidance, ensuring your movements are not only coordinated but also controlled and elegant.

The Joy of Unpredictability: Introducing Challenges

Life is unpredictable, and so is Wall Pilates. In this section, we'll introduce elements of unpredictability to your practice, adding spice to the routine.

Embracing Challenges:

1. Utilizing Props for Variability

Ever tried balancing on one leg while holding a small ball? We'll introduce props and variations to your exercises, turning your routine into an exciting and unpredictable adventure.

2. Adapting to Changing Surfaces

The floor isn't the only stage for Pilates. We'll explore exercises that involve the wall and other surfaces, challenging your balance and coordination in new and exhilarating ways.

3. Embracing Imperfections

Pilates is a journey, not a destination. We'll discuss the beauty of imperfections, emphasizing that stumbling blocks are stepping stones to enhanced balance and coordination.

Case Study: Michael's Success in Preventing Falls

Michael, a lively gentleman in his seventies, had always enjoyed an active

lifestyle. He spent his younger years hiking, playing sports, and dancing, and his zest for life never waned. However, as he aged, he started noticing a gradual decline in his balance and coordination, which raised concerns about his risk of falling.

The fear of falling and its potential consequences, including injuries and loss of independence, troubled Michael. He understood the importance of maintaining his balance, so he began searching for a solution that would allow him to continue enjoying his active life safely.

That's when he was introduced to Wall Pilates, a practice designed to enhance balance and prevent falls among seniors.

Michael's first Wall Pilates class was eye-opening. The instructor explained how the exercises focused on core strength, posture, and coordination, all of which were crucial for maintaining balance and stability. The use of the wall for support was a game-changer for him.

As Michael embarked on his Wall Pilates journey, he was delighted to find that the exercises were not only beneficial but also enjoyable. He felt his strength and balance improving with each session, and the fear of falling began to dissipate. The exercises challenged him, but he embraced the challenge with enthusiasm.

Over time, Michael's balance and coordination reached a level he hadn't experienced in years. The fear of falling no longer controlled his thoughts. He returned to his active lifestyle with newfound confidence, hiking, dancing, and engaging in his favorite activities.

Reflecting on his experience, Michael shared, "Wall Pilates has given me a renewed sense of independence. I can do the things I love without constantly worrying about falling. It's not just about preventing falls; it's about enjoying life to the fullest."

Michael's story underscores the transformative power of Wall Pilates in enhancing balance and preventing falls among seniors. It serves as an inspiring example of how dedicated practice can restore confidence and allow individuals like Michael to embrace an active and fulfilling life with reduced fear of falling.

Studies have shown that Pilates exercise decreases the risk of falls (Pata et al., 2014; Barker et al., 2016; Josephs et al., 2016) and improves functional mobility.

As you immerse yourself in Chapter 5, remember that enhancing balance and coordination is not just about physical prowess; it's about dancing through life with grace and confidence. So, are you ready to pirouette into a world of stability and coordination? Let's waltz together on the path to a more balanced and harmonious you!

7

Pain Management Through Wall Pilates

Way to go, Pilates enthusiast. Welcome to a chapter that's not just about movement; it's a voyage into the soothing seas of pain management through the magic of Wall Pilates. In this exploration, we'll unravel the therapeutic potential of Wall Pilates, discovering how it becomes a gentle balm for persistent aches and discomfort. So, let's embark on this journey towards a pain-free horizon!

Understanding Pain: A Compassionate Prelude

Before we dive into the healing embrace of Wall Pilates, let's take a moment to understand pain – a language your body uses to communicate.

Compassionate Approach to Pain:

1. Differentiating Between Discomfort and Pain

Pilates is designed to challenge, not harm. We'll explore the nuances between discomfort that leads to growth and pain that signals caution, ensuring your practice is both challenging and safe.

2. Listening to Your Body's Signals

Your body is a wise companion. We'll discuss the importance of tuning in, listening to signals, and responding with kindness to ensure your Wall Pilates journey is tailored to your unique needs.

3. The Holistic Approach to Pain Management

Pain isn't just physical; it intertwines with emotions and mental well-being. We'll delve into the holistic nature of pain management, recognizing that Wall Pilates offers not just physical relief but also emotional and mental respite.

Wall Pilates: A Gentle Ally in Pain Management

Now, let's discover how Wall Pilates, with its gentle yet potent movements, becomes a trusted ally in managing and alleviating pain.

The Healing Power of Wall Pilates:

1. Targeted Exercises for Pain Relief

Each Wall Pilates exercise is a tool in your pain management kit. We'll explore specific exercises designed to target common areas of discomfort, offering relief and promoting healing.

2. Enhancing Flexibility for Joint Pain

If joints are creaking, we've got you covered. Wall Pilates is a master at enhancing flexibility. We'll focus on exercises that gently mobilize joints, reducing stiffness and promoting overall joint health.

3. Strengthening Muscles for Back Pain

Ah, the notorious back pain! Fear not; Wall Pilates is here to lend a helping hand. We'll introduce exercises that strengthen the muscles supporting your spine, offering relief to the often-troubled back.

Mindfulness Practices for Pain Relief

Pilates is not just about physical exercises; it's a mindful journey that can alleviate the burden of pain through focused awareness.

Nurturing the Mind-Body Connection:

1. Breath as a Pain-Relief Mechanism

Your breath is a powerful ally in pain management. We'll explore specific breathing techniques that calm your nervous system, providing relief from chronic pain.

2. Mindful Movement for Emotional Well-being

Pain often brings emotional weight. Wall Pilates, with its mindful movement, becomes a therapeutic space where emotional well-being is nurtured alongside physical relief.

3. The Role of Relaxation Techniques

As you recline against the wall, we'll introduce relaxation techniques that ease tension not just in your muscles but also in your mind, creating a sanctuary for pain relief.

Case Study: A Senior's Journey to Pain-Free Living

Meet Grace, at the ripe age of 72, found herself grappling with the wear and tear that often accompanies the golden years. Chronic joint pain, stiffness,

and a decreased range of motion had begun to impede her once-active lifestyle. Frustrated by the limitations imposed by pain, Grace sought a solution that aligned with her age and physical condition.

Introduced to Wall Pilates through a community wellness program, Grace approached her first session with a mix of curiosity and a dash of skepticism. Having experienced various fitness programs that were too intense or unsuitable for her age, she was hopeful but cautious about finding a practice that would cater to her unique needs.

Grace's journey began with addressing age-related aches, particularly in her knees and lower back. The fear of exacerbating the pain initially made her hesitant to engage in physical activities.

Having tried several fitness routines without much success, Grace was initially skeptical about Wall Pilates. Convincing her that this practice would be gentle yet effective required a careful and patient approach.

The beauty of Wall Pilates lies in its adaptability. Grace's instructor tailored exercises to address her specific joint concerns, emphasizing gentle movements that gradually increased in intensity as her comfort level grew.

Wall Pilates introduced Grace to the mindful aspect of the movement. Focused breath work and relaxation techniques became invaluable tools in managing her pain, providing not just physical relief but also a serene space for emotional well-being.

As Grace consistently engaged in Wall Pilates, a remarkable transformation unfolded. Her range of motion increased, and movements that once caused discomfort became more manageable, allowing her to reclaim activities she thought were resigned to the past.

The targeted exercises, combined with the supportive nature of the wall, *contributed to a significant alleviation of chronic pain. Grace found herself experiencing more pain-free days, enhancing her overall quality of life.*

Wall Pilates not only addressed Grace's physical concerns but also reignited her joy in movement. The practice became a source of empowerment, allowing her to navigate daily activities with newfound confidence.

Grace's journey exemplifies the potential of Wall Pilates as a gentle yet powerful avenue for seniors seeking pain relief and enhanced well-being. Her story serves as an inspiration, emphasizing that age is not a barrier to embracing a pain-free and active lifestyle. Grace's transformation is a testament to the adaptability and effectiveness of Wall Pilates in fostering a life of vitality, regardless of age.

Studies have shown Pilates can alleviate chronic pain in most areas of the body. One study (Natour J, Cazotti LA, Ribeiro LH, et al, 2015) stated Pilates improves pain, function, and quality of life in patients.

As you navigate through Chapter 6, remember that pain management through Wall Pilates is not a battle against your body; it's a compassionate collaboration between you and the healing potential within each movement. So, are you ready to sail into the realm of pain relief and rejuvenation? Let's embark on this voyage together!

8

The Mind-Body Connection in Wall Pilates

Ok, Pilates enthusiasts, let's delve deep into the captivating realm where the mind and body entwine like dance partners in the symphony of Wall Pilates. In this chapter, we explore not just the physical exercises but the mindful essence that transforms each movement into a harmonious conversation between your mind and body. Get ready to embark on a journey where every breath, every stretch, and every twist is a step towards a more profound mind-body connection!

The Breath: A Guiding Rhythm

In Wall Pilates, your breath is more than just inhales and exhales; it's the silent conductor orchestrating the movements.

Breath as Your Guiding Force:

1. Rhythmic Breathing Techniques

We'll unravel the art of rhythmic breathing – a dance between inhales and exhales that synchronizes with each movement. Discover how this mindful breath work not only oxygenates your muscles but also serves as a calming cadence for your mind.

2. Connecting Breath to Movement

In Wall Pilates, each movement is a brushstroke in a painting, and your breath colors it with life. Learn how to connect specific breath patterns to different exercises, creating a seamless flow that deepens the mind-body connection.

3. Breath Awareness for Mindfulness

Beyond the physical benefits, breath awareness fosters mindfulness. We'll explore techniques that draw your attention to the present moment, creating a serene space where stress dissipates, and focus intensifies.

Mindful Movement: Beyond the Physical Pose

Pilates is not a mechanical routine; it's a mindful exploration of movement. Let's unlock the secrets of mindful engagement in each pose.

Presence in Every Pose:

1. Conscious Muscle Engagement

Instead of mechanically going through the motions, we'll delve into the concept of conscious muscle engagement. Discover how this mindfulness approach not only refines your movements but also prevents unnecessary strain.

2. Body Scanning for Awareness

Wall Pilates encourages a profound awareness of your body. We'll introduce body scanning techniques – a mindful journey through each muscle group, ensuring that no part of your body is left untouched or unattended.

3. Mindful Transitions Between Poses

The magic of Wall Pilates lies not just in the poses themselves but in the transitions between them. Explore how mindful transitions enhance the fluidity of your practice, turning it into a graceful dance with the wall.

Visualization: Creating Mental Images of Success

Your mind is a powerful architect. Visualization is the tool that shapes the mental blueprint of your success in Wall Pilates.

Visualization Techniques:

1. Envisioning Correct Form

Close your eyes and visualize the perfect execution of a Pilates pose. We'll explore how this mental rehearsal primes your muscles and sets the stage for success, fostering a sense of confidence and mastery.

2. Creating Positive Affirmations

Words have the power to shape reality. Develop positive affirmations related to your Pilates practice, creating a mental dialogue that boosts your confidence and reinforces the mind-body connection.

3. Visualizing Progress and Growth

In the tapestry of Wall Pilates, visualize the thread of progress. Witness how visualizing your journey – from the first tentative movements to the mastery of challenging poses – becomes a motivational force propelling you forward.

Emma's Emotional Healing Through Wall Pilates:

Emma, a senior in her early seventies, had faced her fair share of life's challenges. From the loss of loved ones to personal health struggles, she had carried emotional burdens that weighed heavily on her spirit. These challenges had taken a toll on her mental well-being, leaving her feeling a sense of sadness and melancholy.

In her quest for emotional healing and peace, Emma turned to Wall Pilates as a source of solace. She was drawn to the practice's focus on the mind-body connection, a key element of Wall Pilates that her instructor had emphasized.

As Emma began her Wall Pilates journey, she initially viewed it as a means to improve her physical health. However, what she discovered was far more profound. The exercises were not just about building physical strength; they required mindfulness and a deep connection between her mind and body.

During her practice, Emma found that she could release the emotional weight she had carried for so long. The controlled movements and focused breathing allowed her to let go of the grief and sadness she had been holding onto. It was as if the mind-body connection in Wall Pilates served as a bridge to emotional healing.

Emma recalls, "Wall Pilates was like a therapeutic journey for me. It allowed me to reconnect with my inner self, release the emotional baggage, and find a sense of peace that I hadn't experienced in years."

As Emma continued her Wall Pilates practice, she noticed a transformation not only in her physical health but also in her mental and emotional well-being. The connection between her mind and body grew stronger, and her outlook on life became more positive.

She adds, "It's not just about physical strength; it's about emotional strength.

Wall Pilates helped me heal from the inside out, and I've learned to embrace life with a renewed sense of joy."

Emma's story beautifully exemplifies the profound emotional healing that can be achieved through Wall Pilates. It highlights the therapeutic and holistic benefits of the practice, emphasizing how it can help seniors like Emma find emotional solace and mental well-being, making it not just a physical journey but a deeply transformative and healing one.

As you immerse yourself in Chapter 7, remember that Wall Pilates is not just a physical workout; it's an invitation to dance with mindfulness, to breathe with intention, and to sculpt a harmonious connection between your mind and body. So, are you ready to embrace the mindful magic of Wall Pilates? Let's take this enchanting journey together!

9

Overcoming Challenges and Plateaus

Great start to the trip that is Pilates, let's navigate the sometimes-choppy waters of challenges and plateaus in your Wall Pilates journey.

In this chapter, we'll explore how to steer through obstacles, overcome plateaus, and keep the sails of your enthusiasm billowing. Get ready to weather the storms and emerge stronger and more resilient on the other side!

Understanding Common Challenges: Navigating the Waves

Embarking on a transformative journey isn't always smooth sailing. Let's identify the common challenges you might encounter and how to navigate through them.

Common Challenges at Sea:

1. Physical Discomfort

Feeling a bit sore or encountering mild discomfort is normal, but we'll explore how to differentiate between the discomfort that accompanies growth and the pain that requires caution.

2. Mental Fatigue

The mind is a powerful ally, but it can also be a formidable opponent. Discover strategies to combat mental fatigue, keeping your enthusiasm buoyant even on days when motivation seems to wane.

3. Time Constraints

In the hustle and bustle of life, finding time for your Pilates practice can be a challenge. We'll discuss creative solutions to navigate time constraints, ensuring that your commitment to Wall Pilates remains steadfast.

Strategies for Overcoming Challenges: Charting Your Course

Every storm is an opportunity to showcase your navigation skills. Let's plot a course through challenges, ensuring that your Wall Pilates ship stays on course.

Navigational Strategies:

1. Adaptive Modifications

When faced with physical discomfort or limitations, we'll explore adaptive modifications to exercises. The wall, your trusty companion, can be utilized in various ways to ensure a safe and effective practice.

2. Mindfulness and Relaxation Techniques:

Mental fatigue can be a formidable adversary. Learn to anchor yourself in mindfulness and relaxation techniques, allowing your mind to recharge and approach each session with renewed vigor.

3. Micro-Practices for Time Management:

Short on time? No worries! Discover the power of micro-practices – quick, focused sessions that can be seamlessly integrated into your daily routine, ensuring consistency in your Wall Pilates practice.

Breaking Through Plateaus: Sailing Beyond Still Waters

Plateaus are like still waters that can halt progress. Let's hoist the sails and navigate through plateaus, ensuring a continuous journey of growth.

Strategies for Plateau Navigation:

1. Introduce Variety

Plateaus often arise when routines become monotonous. We'll explore the introduction of variety into your practice – new exercises, different sequences, and creative approaches that reignite the spark.

2. Progressive Challenges

As your strength and flexibility grow, so should the challenges. We'll discuss how to progressively introduce more advanced poses and exercises, ensuring a continuous upward trajectory in your Wall Pilates journey.

3. Goal Setting and Tracking

Set sail with clear goals on the horizon. We'll delve into the importance of goal setting and tracking your progress, providing a navigational map that keeps you focused and motivated.

Robert's Persistence in the Face of Injuries:

Robert, a determined senior in his mid-sixties, had always been an advocate for an active lifestyle. He engaged in sports, hiked challenging terrains, and enjoyed every moment of his adventurous life. However, an unexpected injury threatened to disrupt his active lifestyle.

One day, while hiking in the mountains, Robert experienced a fall that resulted in a serious knee injury. The injury was not only physically painful but also emotionally challenging for someone who had always been active and independent. Robert knew that his journey to recovery would be a challenging one.

His journey toward healing led him to Wall Pilates, where he hoped to regain his strength and mobility. However, he quickly realized that his journey wouldn't be easy. The knee injury limited his movement and made some Wall Pilates exercises initially impossible to perform.

Robert could have easily given up, believing that his active days were behind him. But his determination and resilience pushed him to persist despite the obstacles.

The Wall Pilates instructor, recognizing Robert's predicament, adapted the exercises to accommodate his injury. They focused on gentle movements and stretches that aimed to strengthen the injured knee without causing further harm. The wall provided crucial support, allowing Robert to perform exercises with confidence.

Robert's progress was slow, but his determination was unwavering. Day by day, he pushed through the discomfort and worked on his knee's rehabilitation. His Wall Pilates practice became not just a physical endeavor but also a testament to his mental strength and resolve.

Over time, Robert's knee began to heal, and his strength returned. He regained his mobility, and his overall fitness improved. Wall Pilates had played a crucial role in his journey to recovery, not only physically but emotionally as well. The practice helped him regain his self-confidence and belief in his ability to overcome adversity.

Robert shares, "I could have let my injury define my limitations, but I chose to define my possibilities instead. Wall Pilates was the bridge to my recovery, and it reminded me that persistence and a positive mindset can conquer even the most challenging setbacks."

Robert's story is a powerful example of how persistence and adaptability can lead to remarkable results, even in the face of physical setbacks. It illustrates how Wall Pilates can be a source of recovery and resilience for seniors like Robert, not only physically but also emotionally.

As you navigate through Chapter 8, remember that challenges and plateaus are not roadblocks but opportunities for growth and refinement. With the right strategies and a resilient spirit, your Wall Pilates journey can weather any storm and sail into new horizons of strength and vitality. So, are you ready to chart your course through challenges and plateaus? Let's set sail together!

10

Integrating Wall Pilates into Daily Life

Hello fellow Pilates pioneers! In this chapter, we'll explore the art of seamlessly weaving Wall Pilates into the tapestry of your daily life. It's not just a workout; it's a lifestyle. Let's uncover ways to make Wall Pilates an integral part of your routine, ensuring that the benefits extend beyond the mat and into every facet of your day!

The Power of Consistency: Making it a Habit

They say consistency is the key, and when it comes to Wall Pilates, this adage holds. Let's discover how to transform your Pilates practice from a sporadic event into a daily ritual.

Building the Habit:

1. Setting Realistic Daily Goals

We'll start by setting achievable daily goals, ensuring that your Wall Pilates routine is not overwhelming. Consistency is built on small, sustainable steps.

2. Creating a Dedicated Space

Designate a space in your home for Wall Pilates. It doesn't need to be expansive; even a cozy corner can serve as your personal Pilates haven. This dedicated space becomes a visual cue, signaling to your mind that it's time for your daily practice.

3. Establishing a Routine

Whether it's morning stretches, a lunchtime session, or an evening wind-down, establish a routine that aligns with your daily schedule. Consistency becomes second nature when your Pilates practice becomes an anticipated part of each day.

Incorporating Pilates into Daily Activities: The Seamless Blend

Wall Pilates doesn't need to be confined to the mat. Let's explore how you can infuse Pilates principles into your daily activities, making it a natural and effortless extension of your lifestyle.

Everyday Pilates Integration:

1. Mindful Posture Throughout the Day

From sitting at your desk to standing in line, we'll explore how to maintain a mindful posture. The wall becomes your imaginary ally, supporting your spine and promoting a posture that exudes confidence and strength.

2. Incorporating Micro-Exercises

Discover the art of micro-exercises – subtle movements that can be seamlessly woven into your day. These can range from toe-tapping to shoulder rolls, keeping your muscles engaged even during moments of stillness.

3. Breathwork in Stressful Situations

Pilates breath work is not reserved for the mat. Learn how to integrate calming breaths during stressful situations – in traffic, during a work break, or whenever life throws a curve ball.

Family and Community Involvement: Pilates Together

The joy of Wall Pilates can be contagious. Let's explore ways to involve your family or community, transforming your practice into a shared experience.

Shared Pilates Moments:

1. Family-Friendly Pilates

Introduce simplified Pilates exercises to your family members, creating a bonding activity that promotes health and well-being. The wall becomes a shared support, fostering a sense of unity.

2. Community Pilates Events:

Organize or participate in community Pilates events. Whether it's a park gathering or a virtual session, creating a sense of community amplifies the enjoyment of Wall Pilates and encourages accountability.

3. Pilates Challenges with Friends:

Turn your Pilates practice into a friendly challenge. Share your goals with friends and embark on a collective journey of growth and improvement.

Sarah's Daily Routine of Wall Pilates:

Sarah, a retired senior in her late seventies, was a firm believer in the idea that a healthy and active lifestyle was the key to aging gracefully. She had dabbled in various fitness practices throughout her life but had never found

something that could seamlessly integrate into her daily routine until she discovered Wall Pilates.

For Sarah, Wall Pilates was not just about structured classes; it was a lifestyle. She began her Wall Pilates journey with the intention of incorporating it into her daily activities. She realized that practicing Wall Pilates regularly could help her maintain her mobility, balance, and overall well-being.

Sarah's daily routine was simple yet effective. Each morning, she dedicated a portion of her day to her Wall Pilates practice, turning it into a ritual. She used her bedroom wall, which she had specially adapted for her practice.

Her routine typically began with gentle warm-up exercises, including controlled breathing and stretches. As she progressed, she would move on to more advanced poses and stretches, always focusing on her core strength and balance.

One of her favorite aspects of Wall Pilates was the adaptability of the practice. Sarah used it as a tool for mindfulness and mental well-being as well. She incorporated elements of meditation into her routine, taking moments of stillness and mindfulness between exercises.

Sarah's Wall Pilates practice served as a continuous thread throughout her day. She found herself incorporating Wall Pilates principles into everyday activities, from sitting and standing with proper posture to using her breath to stay centered and calm.

As a result, her body felt stronger, her posture improved, and she enjoyed increased flexibility. More importantly, her daily Wall Pilates routine had a calming and centering effect on her mind, which she believed contributed to her overall emotional well-being.

Sarah reflects, "Wall Pilates isn't just an exercise; it's a way of life. It's a practice that grounds me physically and mentally. I can feel the difference it's made in my overall well-being."

Sarah's story emphasizes the practicality and adaptability of Wall Pilates. It showcases how the practice can become an integral part of a senior's daily routine, contributing to physical well-being and emotional balance. Her experience serves as an inspiring example of how Wall Pilates can be seamlessly integrated into daily life, allowing seniors to age gracefully with a holistic approach to wellness.

As you dive into Chapter 9, remember that Wall Pilates is not a compartmentalized activity; it's a lifestyle that seamlessly blends with the rhythm of your day. By making it an integral part of your routine and involving your loved ones, you transform Pilates from a workout into a joyful and sustainable way of living. So, are you ready to infuse your daily life with the vibrancy of Wall Pilates? Let's embark on this journey of integration together!

11

Celebrating Your Progress and Future Possibilities

Almost done, Pilates trailblazers! As we approach the final chapter of our Wall Pilates odyssey, it's time to bask in the glory of your achievements, acknowledge the journey, and set sail toward the boundless horizons of future possibilities. This chapter is a celebration – a tribute to your commitment, resilience, and the transformative power of Wall Pilates.

Reflecting on Your Pilates Odyssey: The Journey Thus Far

Before we set our sights on the future, let's take a moment to reflect on the path you've traversed. It's a journey marked by dedication, mindful movements, and a growing connection between your mind and body.

Celebrating Milestones:

1. Acknowledge Your Achievements

Take stock of the milestones you've achieved – from mastering challenging poses to cultivating a consistent Pilates routine. Each achievement is a testament to your dedication and progress.

2. Embrace Growth Beyond the Mat

Celebrate not only the physical changes but also the mental and emotional growth. Your journey with Wall Pilates has likely transcended the mat, influencing how you approach challenges, manage stress, and view your overall well-being.

3. Gratitude for the Pilates Community

If you've engaged with a Pilates community or had the support of friends and family, express gratitude for the shared encouragement and inspiration. The community has been a buoyant force on this Pilates voyage.

Setting Sail to Future Possibilities: Charting a Course Forward

As one chapter closes, another beckons. Let's explore the exciting possibilities that lie ahead and how you can continue to evolve on your Wall Pilates journey.

Future Pilates Horizons:

1. Setting New Goals

The beauty of Wall Pilates lies in its adaptability and scalability. Set new goals that challenge and inspire you. Whether it's mastering an advanced pose or deepening your mind-body connection, the horizon is yours to conquer.

2. Exploring Advanced Techniques

With a solid foundation in place, consider exploring advanced Pilates techniques. These may involve incorporating props, trying new sequences, or delving into Pilates fusion practices that blend elements of different movement disciplines.

3. Sharing Your Pilates Wisdom

If you've experienced transformative benefits, consider sharing your Pilates journey with others. Whether through teaching, blogging, or creating social media content, your story has the power to inspire and guide fellow Pilates enthusiasts.

A Heartfelt Pilates Farewell: Navigating Beyond

As we bid adieu to this comprehensive guide on Wall Pilates, remember that your journey is an ongoing exploration. Pilates is not a destination but a lifelong voyage of self-discovery and well-being.

Parting Words of Wisdom:

1. Embrace the Ebb and Flow

Just as the tide ebbs and flows, so does your Pilates journey. Embrace the variations in intensity, the moments of challenge, and the periods of gentle flow. Each phase contributes to your growth.

2. Cultivate Mindful Gratitude

Express gratitude for the benefits – physical, mental, and emotional – that Wall Pilates has bestowed upon you. The wall, your constant companion, has witnessed your triumphs and supported you through challenges.

3. Celebrate Each Practice

Whether it's a quick session or a comprehensive workout, celebrate each practice. Every movement contributes to your well-being, and every moment on the mat is a step towards a healthier and more vibrant you.

William's Remarkable Transformation

William had always been an active individual throughout his life. However, as he approached his seventies, he started to notice the effects of aging on his body. Everyday activities became more challenging, and he began experiencing joint pain and stiffness.

One day, while visiting his local community center, William noticed a group of seniors engaging in a unique form of exercise that piqued his interest – Wall Pilates. He decided to give it a try, albeit with some skepticism.

As William recounts, "I thought, 'Can this really make a difference at my age?' But I was willing to try anything to regain my mobility and live pain-free."

His journey with Wall Pilates began with trepidation. The first few sessions were not easy, and he felt like he was starting from scratch. Yet, he persisted, recognizing that this was a long-term commitment to his health and well-being.

Over time, William started to experience significant improvements. His posture became more upright, and his balance began to stabilize. The chronic joint pain that had once plagued him started to subside. The simple, yet effective Wall Pilates exercises played a pivotal role in this transformation.

He remarks, "I never thought that a few exercises using a wall could have such a profound impact on my life. I feel like I've been given a second chance to enjoy my retirement years to the fullest."

William's story illustrates the transformative power of Wall Pilates, even for seniors who might be initially skeptical or facing physical challenges. It highlights the potential for remarkable progress and lifelong vitality that Wall Pilates offers to those who commit to its practice.

As we conclude this guide, remember that your Pilates adventure is a perpetual expedition filled with joy, discovery, and the promise of continued growth. Celebrate your progress, savor the present, and set sail toward the endless possibilities that await on the horizon. May your Pilates odyssey be everlasting and enriching!

12

Review Request Page

Hey there, Pilates enthusiasts!

We hope you're feeling as fabulous as ever while defying Father Time with your favorite wall exercises. We're reaching out to you, our incredible community, because we value your input and believe your experience with "Senior Wall Pilates: How to Age Gracefully, Increase Flexibility, and Maintain Balance Using a Wall to Defy Father Time" could be a game-changer for others.

So, why should you take a few minutes to leave a review? Well, besides the warm, fuzzy feeling of helping fellow Pilates lovers, your review can make a significant impact on someone else's journey to wellness. Imagine a world where others can age with grace, boost flexibility, and maintain balance just like you. Your review could be the key to unlocking that possibility for them.

Now, let's ponder this: have you ever stumbled upon a book or product that changed your life? Did you wish more people knew about it? Your review can be that guiding light for someone else. It's like passing on the secret to a fulfilling, healthier life - the kind of wisdom that's too good to keep to yourself.

Leaving a review is not just about sharing your thoughts; it's an opportunity to pay it forward. Think about the impact your insights could have on someone who's just starting their Pilates journey or looking for effective ways to age gracefully. Your words might be the encouragement they need to take the first step towards a healthier, happier life.

Now, let's get down to business! We kindly ask you to share your honest thoughts on "Senior Wall Pilates." It's super easy – just head to your favorite online retailer, find the book, and leave a review. Your input can make all the difference for someone deciding whether to embark on this transformative journey.

But wait, there's more! By leaving a review, you're not only helping others but also contributing to the positive energy within our incredible community. It's a win-win situation where everyone benefits from shared experiences and knowledge.

As a thank you, we promise to continue bringing you valuable content and exciting updates on senior Pilates. Your support means the world to us, and we can't wait to see the positive impact your reviews will have on others.

So, what are you waiting for? Help us spread the joy of "Senior Wall Pilates" by leaving your review today. Your words have the power to inspire and guide someone towards a healthier, more balanced life.

Thank you for being an essential part of our community!

Happy reviewing!

13

Conclusion

Embracing the Ageless You

As we draw the curtain on this odyssey through the world of Wall Pilates, it's time to reflect on the profound journey you've undertaken and the ageless version of yourself that has emerged. This conclusion is not just an end but a commencement—a celebration of the vibrant, resilient, and ageless spirit that resides within you.

Reflecting on the Pilates Odyssey: A Tapestry of Growth

You embarked on this Pilates journey with a curiosity to defy Father Time, and along the way, you've woven a tapestry of growth, resilience, and mindful transformation.

Key Reflections:

1. Mind-Body Symbiosis

The essence of Wall Pilates lies not just in the physical movements but in the symbiotic relationship between your mind and body. The journey has deepened your awareness, fostering a connection that transcends the mat.

2. Adaptability and Progress

The adaptability of Wall Pilates allows you to tailor each session to your needs, making progress an organic and enjoyable process. You've witnessed the evolution of your strength, flexibility, and overall well-being.

3. Community and Support

Whether through virtual connections or shared sessions with friends and family, the Pilates community has been a pillar of support. The collective encouragement has added a layer of joy to your journey.

Embracing the Ageless You: A Celebration of Vitality

As you stand at the intersection of the past and the future, it's time to revel in the ageless version of yourself that has blossomed through Wall Pilates.

Key Celebrations:

1. Physical Vitality

Celebrate the newfound vitality in your movements. The strength, flexibility, and balance you've cultivated are not just physical attributes but a testament to the ageless vigor that resides within you.

2. Mindful Resilience

Your journey through challenges and plateaus showcased not only physical resilience but also the mental fortitude to navigate obstacles. The mindful approach to Pilates has become a wellspring of resilience in your daily life.

3. Inspirational Presence

Whether you realize it or not, your commitment to Wall Pilates has become an inspiration to those around you. Your dedication to well-being, the joy you find in movement, and the ageless glow you exude serve as beacons for others on their paths.

The Ongoing Pilates Adventure: A Lifelong Voyage

As we bid farewell to this comprehensive guide, remember that your Pilates adventure is not confined to these pages; it's a lifelong voyage.

Guiding Principles for the Future:

1. Consistent Exploration

Keep exploring the depths of Wall Pilates. The mat is your canvas, and each session is an opportunity to paint new strokes, refine your practice, and uncover uncharted possibilities.

2. Joyful Consistency

Embrace the joy of consistent practice. Whether it's a daily routine or periodic sessions, let the joy of movement be a guiding force, propelling you toward continued growth and well-being.

3. Ageless Mindset

Age is but a number; your vitality is timeless. Embrace the ageless mindset that Wall Pilates has nurtured within you. Every session is a celebration of your ageless spirit.

Epilogue

Sailing into a Timeless Horizon

As the final chapter of this Pilates adventure concludes, envision yourself sailing into a timeless horizon. The wall, a steadfast companion, is not just a support but a witness to the ageless you—an embodiment of strength, vitality, and the perpetual pursuit of well-being.

May your Pilates journey be an everlasting odyssey into the ageless, vibrant, and resilient version of yourself. Let the ageless you continue to flourish with each mindful movement, on and beyond the mat!

14

REFERENCES

1. Kloubec, J. A. (2011). Exploring Pilates: Mechanisms and Recipients. *Muscles, Ligaments and Tendons Journal*, 1(2), 61–66.
2. Barker, A., et al. (2016). Assessing the Feasibility of Pilates Exercise in Reducing Falls Risk: A Preliminary Randomized Controlled Trial in Older Community-Dwellers. *Clinical Rehabilitation*.
3. Pata, R. W., et al. (2014). Enhancing Mobility, Postural Stability, and Balance in Older Adults: A Pilates-Based Exercise Approach. *Journal of Bodywork and Movement Therapies*.
4. Josephs, S., et al. (2016). Pilates for Balance: A Study on its Effectiveness in Preventing Falls among Community-Dwelling Older Adults. *Journal of Bodywork and Movement Therapies*.
5. Natour, J., Cazotti, L. A., Ribeiro, L. H., et al. (2015). Pilates Intervention for Chronic Low Back Pain: A Randomized Controlled Trial on Pain Relief, Function, and Quality of Life. *Clinical Rehabilitation*, 29, 59–68.
6. ChatGPT. (2024). Personalized AI Assistance. *OpenAI*.

15

Wall Pilates Exercises

The following exercises are broken up into categories based on which parts of the body or functionality you are looking to engage. They are Upper Body, Lower Body, Core, Balance and Stability, Mobility, and Flexibility.

Some exercises will fit into more than one category and that is ok. This will allow for more variation and keep workouts from becoming stagnant and repetitious. Mix and match to achieve your individual goals.

16

Wall Pilates for Upper Body

1. Wall Arm Circles

Purpose: Improve shoulder mobility and flexibility.

Instructions:

Stand facing the wall with your feet hip-width apart.

Place your palms flat against the wall at shoulder height.

Begin making slow, controlled circles with your arms, moving them forward and then backward.

Perform 10-15 circles in each direction.

2. Wall Push-Ups

Purpose: Strengthen the chest, shoulders, and triceps.

Instructions:

Stand facing the wall at arm's length.

Place your palms flat against the wall at shoulder height, slightly wider than shoulder width apart.

Step back a bit to create a slight angle.

Keep your body in a straight line and bend your elbows to lower your chest toward the wall.

Push back up to the starting position. Perform 10-15 repetitions.

3. Wall Angels

Purpose: Enhance shoulder mobility and strengthen upper back muscles.

Instructions:

Stand facing the wall with your feet hip-width apart.

Place your back against the wall, ensuring your heels, hips, shoulders, and head all touch the wall.

Raise your arms to shoulder height with your elbows bent at 90 degrees.

Slowly slide your arms up the wall, keeping your elbows and wrists in contact with the wall.

Lower your arms back down to the starting position. Perform 10-15 repetitions.

4. Wall Bicep Curls

Purpose: Strengthen the biceps.

Instructions:

Stand facing the wall with your feet hip-width apart.

Place your palms against the wall at shoulder height.

Bend your elbows to bring your body closer to the wall.

Push away from the wall by straightening your arms. Perform 10-15 repetitions.

5. Wall Triceps Extensions

Purpose: Strengthen the triceps.

Instructions:

Stand facing the wall with your feet hip-width apart.

Place your palms on the wall at shoulder height.

Step back slightly to create tension in your arms.

Bend your elbows to lower your body toward the wall.

Push back up to the starting position. Perform 10-15 repetitions.

6. Wall Shoulder Blade Squeezes

Purpose: Improve upper back strength and posture.

Instructions:

Stand facing the wall with your feet hip-width apart.

Place your palms on the wall at shoulder height.

Squeeze your shoulder blades together as you push your chest toward the wall.

Hold for a few seconds, then relax. Perform 10-15 repetitions

7. Wall Y-Raises

Purpose: Strengthen the upper back, and shoulders, and improve posture.

Instructions:

Stand facing the wall with your feet hip-width apart.

Extend your arms straight out in a Y-shape, with your palms flat against the wall at shoulder height.

Gently push into the wall and squeeze your shoulder blades together.

Hold for a few seconds, then relax. Perform 10-15 repetitions.

8. Wall Chest Opener

Purpose: Stretch and open the chest and shoulders.

Instructions:

Stand facing the wall with your feet hip-width apart.

Place your palms on the wall at chest height, with your fingers pointing downward.

Gently lean forward, feeling a stretch across your chest and shoulders.

Hold the stretch for 20-30 seconds. Repeat the stretch 2-3 times.

17

Wall Pilates for Lower Body

1. Wall Squats

Purpose: Strengthening the quadriceps and glutes while improving balance.

Instructions:

Stand with your back against the wall, feet hip-width apart.

Slowly slide down the wall, bending your knees and hips as if you're sitting in a chair.

Keep your back against the wall and ensure your knees don't go beyond your toes.

Hold this position for 10-15 seconds, or as long as you're comfortable.

Slowly return to the starting position.

2. Wall Leg Raises

Purpose: Enhancing hip and thigh strength and improving balance.

Instructions:

Stand facing the wall with your hands lightly touching it for balance.

Lift one leg to the side as high as you comfortably can, keeping it straight.

Hold the leg in the raised position for a few seconds.

Slowly lower the leg back to the ground.
Repeat on the other leg.

3. Wall Calf Raises

Purpose: Strengthening the calf muscles and improving ankle stability.

Instructions:

Stand facing the wall with your hands lightly touching it for support.

Lift your heels off the ground as high as you comfortably can, rising onto your toes.

Hold this position for a few seconds.

Lower your heels back to the ground. Repeat the movement.

4. Wall Leg Swings

Purpose: Improving hip flexibility and leg mobility.

Instructions:

Stand facing the wall, placing your hands lightly against it for balance.
Swing one leg forward and backward in a controlled manner.
Aim for a gentle and controlled range of motion.
After several swings, switch to the other leg.

5. Wall Lunges

Purpose: Strengthening the quadriceps, hamstrings, and glutes while improving balance.

Instructions:

Stand with your back against the wall, feet hip-width apart.
Take a step forward with one foot, bending both knees to create a lunge position.
Make sure your front knee doesn't go beyond your toes.
Hold the lunge position for a few seconds.
Return to the starting position and repeat on the other leg.

6. Wall Sitting Leg Lifts

Purpose: Enhancing thigh and hip strength.

Instructions:

Sit against the wall with your legs extended in front of you.

Lift one leg as high as you comfortably can while keeping it straight.

Hold this position for a few seconds.

Lower the leg and switch to the other leg.

18

Wall Pilates for Core Strength

1. Wall Sit with Pelvic Tilts:

Stand with your back against the wall and lower yourself into a seated position.
   Perform gentle pelvic tilts, engaging your core muscles.

2. Wall Squats:

Stand with your back against the wall and lower into a squat position.
   Hold the squat, engage your core, and then return to the starting position.

3. Wall Plank:

Place your hands on the wall at shoulder height.
   Step back to create a straight line from head to heels, engaging your core.

4. Wall Leg Lifts:

Stand facing the wall with your hands on it for support.

Lift one leg straight out in front of you, engaging your core.

Lower the leg and repeat on the other side.

5. Wall Bridge:

Lie on your back with your feet against the wall and knees bent.

Lift your hips towards the ceiling, engaging your core and squeezing your glutes.

6. Wall Knee Tucks:

Start in a plank position facing the wall.

Bring one knee towards your chest and then switch legs, keeping your core tight.

7. Wall Roll-Downs:

Stand with your back against the wall and slowly roll down, articulating your spine.

Engage your core as you roll back up.

8. Wall Side Plank:

Lie on your side with your elbow directly under your shoulder and your feet against the wall.

Lift your hips, creating a straight line from head to feet.

9. Wall Crunches:

Lie on your back with your feet against the wall and knees bent.

Perform small crunches, engaging your core without straining your neck.

10. Wall Rotation:

Sit on the floor with your side against the wall, knees bent.
Rotate your torso towards the wall, engaging your obliques.

19

Wall Pilates for Balance and Stability

1. Wall Leg Lifts:
Stand facing a wall with your hands lightly resting on the wall for support.
Lift one leg slightly off the ground and hold it in the air for a few seconds.
Slowly lower the leg and repeat on the other side.
Aim to increase the duration of the leg lift as your balance improves.

2. Wall Squats:
Stand with your back against the wall and your feet shoulder-width apart.
Slowly lower your body into a squat position, as if you were sitting in an invisible chair.
Keep your back against the wall and your knees in line with your ankles.
Hold the squat position for a few seconds and then stand back up.
Repeat this exercise for a designated number of repetitions.

3. Wall Marching:
Stand facing the wall with your hands lightly touching it for support.
Lift one knee as high as you can while balancing on the other leg.
Hold the raised knee for a few seconds, then lower it and switch to the other leg.

Continue marching in place against the wall.

4. Wall Planks:

Place your hands on the wall at shoulder height, with your arms fully extended.

Step your feet back so your body forms a straight line from head to heels.

Engage your core and hold the position for as long as you can.

Gradually increase the duration of the plank as your strength and balance improve.

5. Wall Tap and Reach:

Stand facing the wall with your hands lightly touching it.

Lift one leg and tap your toe to the side, then return to the center.

Next, reach the same leg behind you and tap your toes, then return to the center.

Continue alternating between tapping to the side and reaching behind with each leg.

6. Wall Tai Chi Leg Swing:

Stand next to the wall with your fingertips lightly touching for support.

Swing one leg forward and backward in a controlled motion.

Focus on balance as you swing your leg, keeping your core engaged.

Switch to the other leg and repeat.

7. Wall Tree Pose:

Stand with your side to the wall and place one foot against your inner thigh.

Press your hands together in front of your chest in a prayer position.

Hold this tree pose for balance, ensuring your foot is pressing firmly against your inner thigh.

These exercises are tailored to help seniors improve their balance and stability while providing the necessary support and safety.

20

Wall Pilates for Mobility

Section 1: Neck and Shoulder Mobility

1. Neck Rolls

Stand with your back to the wall and your feet hip-width apart.

Gently drop your chin to your chest and slowly roll your head from side to side.

Perform this motion for 30 seconds, focusing on the flexibility of your neck.

2. Shoulder Blade Squeezes

Stand with your back against the wall, keeping your feet a few inches away.

Lift your arms to shoulder height, bend your elbows at 90 degrees, and press them against the wall.

Squeeze your shoulder blades together for 10 seconds, then release.

Repeat this exercise 10 times.

3. Arm Circles

Stand with your feet hip-width apart, facing the wall.

Place your hands on the wall at shoulder height.

Begin making small clockwise circles with your hands.

After 20 seconds, switch to counterclockwise circles.

Repeat the process for 2 minutes, gradually extending the circle size.

Section 2: Hip and Knee Mobility

1. Wall Hip Flexor Stretch

Stand facing the wall, about an arm's length away.

Lift one knee and place your foot flat against the wall.

Gently lean your weight forward to feel a stretch in your hip flexor.

Hold for 20-30 seconds on each side, breathing deeply.

2. Wall Leg Swings

Stand sideways to the wall, using one hand for support.

Swing one leg forward and backward while keeping it straight.

Perform 10 swings on each leg, gradually increasing the range of motion.

3. Wall Squats for Knee Mobility

Stand with your back against the wall and your feet about hip-width apart.

Slowly slide down the wall into a squatting position, keeping your knees aligned with your feet.

Hold the squat for 10 seconds, then push yourself back up.

Repeat this exercise 10 times.

Section 3: Spinal Mobility

1. Wall Cat-Cow Stretch

Face the wall and place your hands on it at shoulder height.
Inhale, arch your back and look up (Cow Pose).
Exhale, round your back, and tuck your chin to your chest (Cat Pose).
Repeat this sequence for 1 minute, focusing on spinal flexibility.

2. Wall Rotations

Stand facing the wall, arms extended at shoulder height.
Rotate your upper body to one side, keeping your feet planted.
Return to the center and repeat the rotation to the other side.
Perform 10 rotations on each side.

3. Wall Hamstring Stretch

Stand facing the wall with your feet hip-width apart.
Extend one leg straight in front of you and place your heel on the wall.
Gently lean forward to feel a stretch in your hamstring.
Hold for 20-30 seconds on each leg.

Section 4: Ankle and Foot Mobility

1. Wall Ankle Circles

Stand facing the wall with your feet hip-width apart.
Lift one foot off the ground and rotate your ankle in a circular motion.
Perform 10 circles clockwise, then 10 circles counterclockwise, and switch to the other foot.

2. Wall Calf Stretch

Stand facing the wall and place your hands on it for support.

Step one foot back and press your heel into the ground.

Keep your back leg straight and bend your front knee slightly to feel the stretch in your calf.

Hold for 20-30 seconds on each leg.

3. Wall Toe Taps

Sit on a chair or stool with your feet flat on the ground.

Place a small object (e.g., a tennis ball) on the floor in front of you.

Use your toes to tap the object repeatedly, working on your toe mobility.

Perform this exercise for 2 minutes.

Section 5: Hand and Wrist Mobility

1. Wall Wrist Flexor Stretch

Stand facing the wall with your arm extended in front of you, palm facing the wall.

Gently press your fingers against the wall and lean your body forward.

Feel the stretch in your wrist and forearm.

Hold for 20-30 seconds on each arm.

2. Wall Finger Taps

Stand facing the wall with your arm extended in front of you, fingers touching the wall.

Begin tapping your fingers against the wall, working on finger mobility.

Perform this exercise for 2 minutes.

3. Wall Hand Circles

Stand facing the wall and place your palms flat against it.

Make circles with your hands in both directions, focusing on wrist and hand flexibility.

Perform this exercise for 1-2 minutes.

21

Wall Pilates for Flexibility

1. Wall Stretch and Reach:

Stand facing the wall, about an arm's length away.

Place your hands flat against the wall at shoulder height.

Slowly walk your hands up the wall while keeping your feet in place.

As you walk your hands up, reach your body forward, feeling the stretch in your shoulders and spine.

Hold for 20-30 seconds, then walk your hands back down.

2. Wall Leg Stretch:

Stand facing the wall with your hands resting on it for support.

Lift one leg and press the sole of your foot against the wall.

Gently push your foot into the wall to feel a stretch in your hamstrings and calf.

Hold for 20-30 seconds, then switch to the other leg.

3. Wall Assisted Forward Bend:

Stand facing the wall and place your hands against it at chest height.

Step back a few feet and keep your feet hip-width apart.

Bend at your hips and let your body hang forward, maintaining contact with the wall for support.

Allow your back to lengthen and your spine to stretch.

Hold for 20-30 seconds, breathing deeply.

4. Wall Hip Flexor Stretch:

Stand with your side facing the wall.

Place one hand on the wall for balance.

Take a step back with your outside leg and bend your front knee to a 90-degree angle.

Feel the stretch in the hip flexor of your back leg.

Hold for 20-30 seconds, then switch sides.

5. Wall Quadriceps Stretch:

Stand with your side facing the wall.

Place one hand on the wall for balance.

Bend your outside knee and reach behind to grab your ankle.

Gently pull your heel toward your buttocks to stretch your quadriceps.

Hold for 20-30 seconds, then switch legs.

6. Wall Shoulder Opener:

Stand facing the wall and place your hands against it at shoulder height.

Walk your feet back and lower your chest towards the floor, keeping your arms straight.

Feel the stretch in your shoulders and chest.

Hold for 20-30 seconds, then slowly walk your feet back in.

7. Wall Arm Circles:

Stand facing the wall, with your palms resting against it at shoulder height.

Begin making small circles with your arms in a forward direction.

Gradually increase the size of the circles, feeling the stretch in your shoulder and chest.

After a few rotations, switch to backward circles. Continue for 20-30 seconds in each direction.

8. Wall Cat-Cow Stretch:

Stand with your side facing the wall.

Place one hand on the wall for balance.

Bend your knees slightly and round your back, like a "cat."

Then, arch your back, sticking your buttocks out, like a "cow."

Move through these two positions slowly, emphasizing the stretch in your spine.

Repeat for 20-30 seconds, then switch sides.

9. Wall Pilates Mermaid Stretch:

Sit on the floor with your side against the wall.

Extend your legs in a straddle position.

Place your hand on the wall and lean gently in the opposite direction.

Feel the stretch along your side and oblique muscles.

Hold for 20-30 seconds, then switch sides.

10. Wall Hip Opener and Stretch:

Stand facing the wall, with your hands on the wall for support.

Lift one knee and gently rotate it outward, creating a 90-degree angle with your hip and knee.

Feel the stretch in your hip joint and groin area.

IIold for 20-30 seconds, then switch to the other leg.

11. Wall Relaxation and Mindfulness:

Sit or lie down with your back against the wall.

Close your eyes and focus on your breath, inhaling and exhaling slowly and deeply.

Use this time for relaxation, mindfulness, and reducing stress. Practice for 5-10 minutes.

These exercises focus on enhancing flexibility in different areas of the body.

22

EXAMPLE WORK OUT SCHEDULE

SENIOR WALL PILATES

<u>USE EXERCISES FROM ALL 6 CATEGORIES</u>

UPPER BODY   LOWER BODY   CORE   BALANCE AND STABILITY   MOBILITY

FLEXIBILTY

SOME EXERCISES FALL INTO MORE THAN ONE CATEGORY

HERE IS AN EXAMPLE PROGRAM

Sunday	Monday	Tuesday	Wednesday	Thursday	Friday	Saturday
	1 1-Upper Body 1-Lower Body	2	3 1-Upper Body 1-Lower Body	4	5 1-Upper Body 1-Lower Body	6
7	8 1-Upper Body 1-Lower Body	9	10 1-Upper Body 1-Lower Body	11	12 1-Upper Body 1-Lower Body	13
14	15 2-Upper Body 2-Lower Body	16 1- Core/Mobility 1-Flexiblity	17 2-Upper Body 2-Lower Body	18 1-Core/Mobility 1-Balance	19 2-Upper Body 2-Lower Body	20
21	22 2-Upper Body 2-Lower Body	23 2-Core/Mobility 2-Flexiblity	24 2-Upper Body 2-Lower Body	25 2-Balance/Stability 2-Flexiblity	26 2-Upper Body 2-Lower Body	27
28	29 2-Upper Body 2-Lower Body	30 2-Core/Mobility 2-Flexiblity	31 2-Upper Body 2-Lower Body	1 2-Balance/Stability 2-Flexiblity	2 2-Upper Body 2-Lower Body	3
4	5 3-Upper Body 3-Lower Body	6 3-Balance/Stability 2-Flexiblity	7 3-Upper Body 3-Lower Body	8 3-Balance/Stability 2-Core	9 3-Upper Body 3-Lower Body	10 2-Core 2-Flexiblity

STEADY PROGRESSION
MIX AND MATCH
CATEGORIES TO KEEP
WORKOUTS FRESH

Building to a Lifestyle

Wall Pilates should become part of your daily routine. Eventually getting to 7 days a week with a mixture of Upper, Lower, Core, Flexibility, Mobility, Stability, and Relaxation Exercises.

Individual Programs

Based on your mobility, flexibility, and range of motion. You can create your own program that will keep the routine fresh and engaging. Be Creative.

Sundays

Will eventually become the Mind-Body connection day. With emphasis on breathing and meditation to focus the mind and body for the next week's workout.